THE SAW PALMETTO STORY:
Nature's Answer to Prostate Enlargement

Table of Contents

Introduction

Saw palmetto *(Serenoa repens)*, a small palm tree native to the Atlantic Coast of North America from South Carolina to Florida, may provide the answer to a common ailment among men. Based on current scientific knowledge, the fat-soluble (liposterolic) extract of the berries from this plant offers nature's most effective remedy for an enlarged prostate.

The prostate—a single, doughnut-shaped gland about the size of a chestnut—lies below the bladder and surrounds the urethra. The prostate gland secretes fluids which lubricate the urethra and increase sperm motility. Prostatic secretions account for about 30% of the volume of semen.

Nearly 60% of men aged 40 to 59 have an enlarged prostate gland, a condition known in the medical community as **benign prostatic hyperplasia** (BPH, formerly known as benign prostatic hypertrophy).[1] The cost of hospital care and surgery for BPH in the United States alone is over one billion dollars each year.[2]

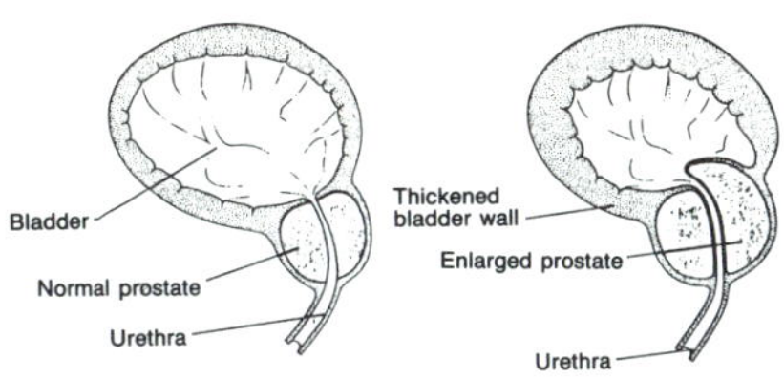

An enlarged prostate can block the urethra, reducing the flow of urine.

BPH symptoms typically reflect blockage of the bladder outlet (progressive frequency and urgency of urination; waking during the night to empty the bladder; hesitancy and intermittency with reduced force and caliber of urine).

If left untreated, the condition may block the bladder outlet completely, causing urine retention in the blood (uremia).

Please Note: Benign Prostatic Hyperplasia can only be diagnosed by a physician. Do not self-diagnose. If you are experiencing any symptoms associated with BPH, see your physician immediately for proper diagnosis.

Many physicians feel surgery is the only solution to the problem. An effective and safe alternative is desperately needed because the surgical procedure often results in significant complications. The fat-soluble extract of saw palmetto berries may provide this safe and effective alternative.

What Causes BPH?

Altered Hormone Levels

As men age, their hormone levels change.[2] Testosterone and, in particular, free testosterone levels decrease after the fifth decade of life. The levels actually increase for other hormones, such as:

- prolactin
- estradiol
- sex hormone-binding ligand
- luteinizing hormone
- follicle-stimulating hormone.

These changes create an increased amount of dihydrotestosterone within the prostate. **Dihydrotestosterone** is a very potent androgen (male hormone) derived from testosterone. It causes the overproduction or hyperplasia of prostate cells which ultimately results in prostate enlargement.

Dihydrotestosterone levels increase within prostate cells due to three reasons:

1) a greater uptake of testosterone,
2) a much higher activity of the enzyme which converts testosterone to dihydrotestosterone, and
3) a lower rate of breakdown and excretion of dihydrotesterone.[2]

Increased Uptake of Hormones

The increased uptake of testosterone by the prostate appears to be the result of yet another hormone, **prolactin**, secreted by the pituitary gland in the brain. Prolactin also increases the activity of the enzyme which converts testosterone to dihydrotestosterone.

Beer and stress cause increased prolactin levels. These factors may contribute greatly to benign prostatic hyperplasia. Drugs that reduce prolactin levels can reduce many BPH symptoms, but these drugs have severe side effects and are not widely used.

On the other hand, studies show vitamin B6 and the trace mineral zinc can reduce prolactin levels as well, without producing side effects at prescribed doses.[3,4] Zinc and vitamin B6 are intricately involved in hormone metabolism, so a lack of one or both of these nutrients may also contribute to BPH.[5]

Decreased Ability to Break Down Hormones

In addition, prostate cells lose their ability to break down and excrete hormones. Normally, enzymes convert testosterone and dihydrotestosterone to compounds with a low attraction for molecules in the cells that bind these hormones. The metabolized hormones can then be excreted.

When testosterone and dihydrotestosterone are not metabolized and excreted properly, their levels increase dramatically within prostate cells.

The Treatment of BPH

Treatment of BPH must affect the hormonal factors causing increased dihydrotestosterone levels within the prostate. Several treatment measures can significantly reduce dihydrotestosterone levels in the prostate, thus reducing the signs and symptoms of BPH.

SAW PALMETTO *(Serenoa repens)*

History:

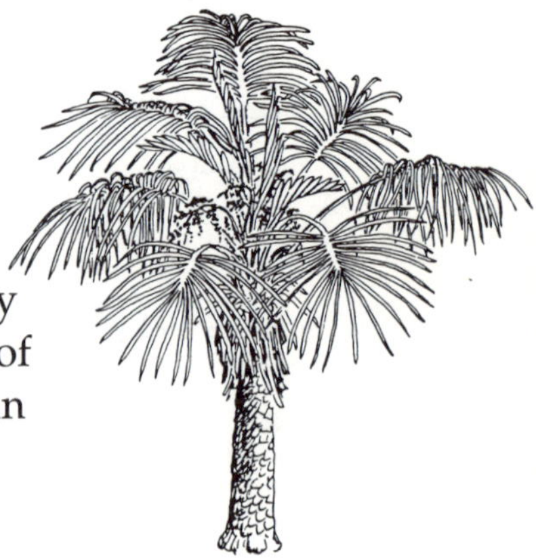

Originally, the American Indians consumed saw palmetto berries as part of their diet. Later, naturopathic physicians also used saw palmetto as a tonic to naturally support the body in the treatment of genito-urinary tract disturbances, in men to increase testicle function, and in women with mammary gland disorders. Many herbalists have regarded it as a mild aphrodisiac.[6]

These historical uses prompted European researchers to investigate the clinical use of saw palmetto berry extracts in BPH. They discovered the fat and sterol portion of the berry offers the greatest therapeutic benefit in treating BPH. A standardized extract of the fat-soluble (liposterolic) fraction of the berries has shown remarkably consistent pharmacological effects.[6-9]

Description:

The saw palmetto grows six to ten feet high with a crown of large leaves. The berries vary in color from deep red-brown to black. They are wrinkled and oblong, ranging in length from one-half to one inch with a diameter of half an inch.[6]

Chemical composition:

Saw palmetto berries contain about 1.5% oil made up of saturated and unsaturated fatty acids and sterols.[6] About 63% of the oil is composed of free fatty acids. The rest contains ethyl esters of these fatty acids and sterols, including beta-sitosterol and its glucoside. The berries also contain carotenes, lipase, tannins, and sugars.

The soluble lipid compounds (fats and oils) are thought to be the major pharmacological components. The purified fat-soluble extract used in treating BPH contains not less than 85% and not more than 95% fatty acids and sterols. This extract contains a complex mixture of saturated and unsaturated free fatty acids (approximately 85%), their methyl- and ethyl-esters (approximately 7%), long-chain alcohols in free and esterified form and various free and esterified sterol derivatives.[6]

Gas chromatography and mass spectrometry have identified the following free fatty acids in this extract:

- capronic acid (C6)
- capric acid (C8)
- caprylic acid (C10)
- lauric acid (C12)
- mirystic acid (C14)

continued on page 10

Table 1. Clinical Studies Demonstrating th

Authors	Type of Study	Number of Patients	Length of Study
Boccafoschi, et al.	Double blind, placebo	22	60 days
Cirillo, et al.	Open	47	4 months
Tripodi, et al.	Open	40	30-90 days
Emili, et al.	Double blind, placebo	30	30 days
Greca, et al.	Open	14	1-2 months
Duvia, et al.	Controlled trial vs. Pygeum africanum	30	30 days
Tamca, et al.	Double blind, placebo	30	31-90 days
Cukier, et al.	Double blind, placebo	168	60-90 days
Champault, et al.	Double blind, placebo	168	60-90 days
Crimi, et al.	Open	32	4 weeks
Champault, et al.	Double blind, placebo	110	28 days

*** DAILY DOSAGE 320 MG.**

Dosage:

The recommended dosage for a liposterolic extract of saw palmetto berries containing 85-95% fatty acids and sterols is 320 mg. per day (160 milligrams twice daily is best). A similar dose using the crude berries would require

Effectiveness of Serenoa Repens* in BPH

Results
Significant difference for: volume voided, maximum flow, mean flow, dysuria, nocturia
Significant difference for: dysuria, nocturia, urine flow
Significant difference for: dysuria, nocturia, volume of prostate, voiding rate, residual urine
Significant difference for: number of voidings
Significant difference for: dysuria, perineal heaviness, nocturia, volume of urine per voiding, interval between two diurnal voidings, sensation of incomplete voiding
Significant difference for: voiding rate
Significant difference for: frequency, urine flow measurement
Significant difference for: dysuria, frequency, residuile urine
Significant difference for: objective and subjective parameters
Significant difference for: dysuria, nocturia, volume of prostate, voiding rate
Significant difference for: dysuria, nocturia, flow measurement, residual urine

at least 10 to 20 grams twice daily. Proper dosages for fluid extracts and tinctures would involve the consumption of extremely large quantities of alcohol; therefore, they cannot be recommended.[6]

- isomirystic acid (C14)
- palmitic acid (C16)
- oleic acid (C18:1)
- stearic acid (C18).

Also, lauric and mirystic acid make up about 30% of the fatty acid content.

The identified alcohols in the saw palmetto berry extract include those with 22, 23, 24, 26, 28, and 30 carbon chains, phytol, farnesol and geranylgeraniol, plus high molecular-weight unsaturated polyprenols.

The sterolic fraction is composed of beta-sitosterol, stigmasterol, cycloartenol, lupeol, lupenone, and 24-methylcycloartenol. Many of these sterols are esterified with the fatty acids of the extract.

Clinical use:

Serenoa repens berries (specifically the fat-soluble extract) are now mainly used in the treatment of benign prostatic hyperplasia.[6]

As detailed earlier, BPH is thought to be caused when testosterone levels build up in the prostate. Within the prostate, testosterone is converted to an even more potent compound called dihydrotestosterone. This compound causes cells to multiply excessively, eventually leading to prostate enlargement.

Studies have shown the fat-soluble saw palmetto berry extract prevents the conversion of testosterone to dihydrotestosterone. It also inhibits dihydrotestosterone's binding to cellular and nuclear receptor sites, thereby increasing the breakdown and excretion of dihydrotestosterone.[6,7,8] Researchers believe these effects are responsible for the impressive clinical results obtained with the liposterolic saw palmetto extract.[9-19]

These positive results on the major symptoms of BPH have been confirmed in several double-blind, placebo-controlled clinical trials.[9-19] (See Table 1 on pages 8 and 9)

Champault, et al. obtained impressive clinical results in their study of 110 outpatients suffering from BPH.[19] In the group receiving the serenoa extract, nighttime urination (number of times) decreased more than 45%, flow rate (ml/s) increased more than 50%, and post-micturition residue (ml) decreased 42%. Those on placebo showed no significant improvement in nocturia or flow rate, and actually worsened in post-micturition residue.

Significant improvements were also noted in self-rating by the patients and global rating by the physician. Of the 50 subjects completing the 30-day study who had taken the liposterolic extract of serenoa, physician's rating noted 14 had improved greatly, 31 had improved somewhat, and only 5 had remained unchanged or worsened.

In contrast, no subjects in the placebo group had greatly improved, 16 experienced some improvement, and 28 remained unchanged or worsened.

These results, combined with those detailed in Table 1, show the liposterolic extract of saw palmetto berries is quite effective in treating BPH.

Toxicity:

No significant side effects have been reported in the clinical trials of the saw palmetto berry extract, or with saw pametto berry ingestion. Toxicology studies in animals have also demonstrated the fat-soluble saw palmetto berry extract produces no side effects.[6]

Summary

Benign prostatic hyperplasia represents a major medical problem in the United States. Each year, over $1 billion is spent on hospital care and surgery for this condition. The standardized fat-soluble extract of saw palmetto berries may offer an effective alternative to surgery.

References

1. Hinman F: Benign Prostatic Hyperplasia. Springer-Verlag, New York, 1983

2. Horton R: Benign prostatic hyperplasia: A disorder of androgen metabolism in the male. J Am Geri Soc 32:380-5, 1984

3. Judd AM, MacLeod RM, and Login IS: Zinc acutely, selectively and reversibly inhibits pituitary prolactin secretion. Brain Res 294:190-2, 1984

4. Vescovi PP, Gerra G, Rastelli G, et al: Pyridoxine (vit. B6) decreases opiods-induced hyperprolactinemia. Horm Metabol Res 17:46-7, 1985

5. Fahim M, Fahim Z, Der R, and Harman J: Zinc treatment for the reduction of hyperplasia of the prostate. Fed Proc 35:361, 1976

6. Pizzorno JE and Murray MT: A Textbook of Natural Medicine. JBC Publications, Seattle, WA, 1989, Chapter V:Serenoa Repens

7. Carilla E, Briley M, Fauran F, et al: Binding of Permixon, a new treatment for prostatic benign hyperplasia, to the cytosolic androgen receptor in the rat prostate. J Steroid Biochem 20:521-3, 1984

8. Sultan C, Terraza A, Devillier C, et al: Inhibition of androgen metabolism and binding by a liposterolic extract of "Serenoa repens B" in human foreskin fibroblasts. J Steroid Biochem 20:515-9, 1984

9. Boccafoschi and Annoscia S: Comparison of Serenoa repens extract with placebo by controlled clinical trial in patients with prostatic adenomatosis. Urologia 50:1257-68, 1983

10. Cirillo-Marucco E, Pagliarulo A, Tritto G, et al: Extract of Serenoa repens (PermixonR) in the early treatment of prostatic hypertrophy. Urologia 5:1269-77, 1983

11. Tripodi V, Giancaspro M, Pascarella M, et al: Treatment of prostatic hypertrophy with Serenoa repens extract. Med Praxis 4:41-6, 1983

12. Emili E, Lo Cigno M and Petrone U: Clinical trial of a new drug for treating hypertrophy of the prostate (Permixon). Urologia 50:1042-8, 1983

13. Greca P and Volpi R: Experience with a new drug in the medical treatment of prostatic adenoma. Urologia 52:532-5, 1985

14. Duvia R, Radice GP and Galdini R: Advances in the phytotherapy of prostatic hypertrophy. Med Praxis 4:143-8, 1983

15. Tasca A, Barulli M, Cavazzana A, et al: Treatment of obstructive symptomatology caused by prostatic adenoma with an extract of Serenoa repens. Double-blind clinical study vs. placebo. Minerva Urol Nefrol 37:87-91, 1985

16. Cukier (Paris), Ducassou (Marseille), Le Guillou (Bordeaux), et al: Permixon versus placebo. C R Ther Pharmacol Clin 4/25:15-21, 1985
17. Champault G, Patel JC and Bonnard AM: A double-blind trial of an extract of the plant Serenoa repens in benign prostatic hyperplasia. Br J Clin Pharmacol 18:461-2, 1984
18. Crimi A and Russo A: Extract of Serenoa repens for the treatment of the functional disturbances of prostate hypertrophy. Med Praxis 4:47-51, 1983
19. Champault G, Bonnard AM, Cauquil J and Patel JC: Medical treatment of prostatic adenoma. Controlled trial: PA 109 vs placebo in 110 patients. Ann Urol 18:407-10, 1984

Vital Communications
THE HEALTH SERIES

by Dr. Michael Murray, N.D.

Includes other unique and interesting booklets on the following subjects:

Alzheimer's Disease
Irritable Bowel Syndrome
Liver Support
Peptic Ulcer
Stress Management

For more information contact:

Vital Communications, Inc
12819 SE 38th St.
Suite 159
Bellevue, WA 98006